Nature's Cure

50 Natural Remedies for Joint Pain Relief"

Copyright

Table Of Content

•Echinacea
•Ginkgo biloba
•Milk thistle
•Holy basil
•Licorice root
•Wild yam
•Birch leaf
•Nettle leaf
•Yucca root
•Calendula
•Sarsaparilla
•Dandelion root
•Cat's claw
•Garlic
•Apple cider vinegar
•Lemon juice
•Aloe vera
•Coconut oil
•Olive oil
•Flaxseed oil
•Fish oil
•Evening primrose oil

•Burdock root
•Red clover
•Meadowsweet
•Valerian root
•Blackcurrant seed oil
•Celery seed oil
•Frankincense oil
•Peppermint oil

Introduction

Joint pain is a common ailment that affects millions of people worldwide. It can be caused by a variety of factors including injury, disease, and aging, and can greatly impact one's quality of life. Many people turn to conventional treatments such as medication and surgery to alleviate their joint pain, but there are also a number of natural remedies that have been used for centuries to alleviate joint pain and inflammation. This book, "Joint Relief: A Comprehensive Guide to Natural Remedies for Joint Pain and Inflammation", is a comprehensive guide to these traditional remedies.

The book covers 50 natural remedies, including herbs, supplements, and oils that have been used to alleviate joint pain and inflammation. Each remedy is thoroughly explained, including its traditional uses, possible side effects, and suggested dosages. The book also includes information on how to use these remedies in conjunction with conventional treatments and tips for maintaining a healthy lifestyle to support joint health.

This book is intended for anyone who is suffering from joint pain and is looking for natural alternatives to conventional treatments. It is designed to be an easy-to-read and informative guide that provides a wealth of information on natural remedies for joint pain and inflammation. Whether you are suffering from osteoarthritis, rheumatoid arthritis, or another joint condition, this book will provide you with the information you need to make informed decisions about your health.

Natural Remedies for Joint Pain

Joint pain is a common ailment that affects people of all ages. In this notebook, we will discuss 50 natural remedies that have been traditionally used to alleviate joint pain and inflammation.

Turmeric: This spice has anti-inflammatory properties and has been used for centuries to treat joint pain. Curcumin, the active ingredient in turmeric, has been shown to reduce inflammation and improve mobility in people with osteoarthritis. You can take turmeric supplements or add the spice to your food.

Ginger: Another anti-inflammatory spice, ginger has been used to treat joint pain for centuries. It contains compounds called gingerols and shogaols that have been shown to reduce inflammation and pain. You can take ginger supplements or add fresh or powdered ginger to your food.

Omega-3 fatty acids: These healthy fats, found in fish such as salmon and mackerel, have anti-inflammatory properties that can help reduce joint pain. Omega-3 supplements are available, or you can get your omega-3s by eating fish or taking fish oil supplements.

Boswellia: This herb, also known as Indian frankincense, has been used in Ayurvedic medicine to treat joint pain and inflammation. It contains compounds called boswellic acids that have been shown to reduce inflammation and improve mobility in people with osteoarthritis.

Glucosamine: This compound, found naturally in the body, is a building block of cartilage. Glucosamine supplements have been shown to reduce pain and improve mobility in people with osteoarthritis.

Chondroitin: This compound, also found naturally in the body, is a component of cartilage. Chondroitin supplements have been shown to reduce pain and improve mobility in people with osteoarthritis.

Bromelain: This enzyme, found in pineapple, has anti-inflammatory properties and has been used to treat joint pain. Bromelain supplements are available, or you can eat fresh pineapple.

Devil's claw: This herb, native to southern Africa, has been used to treat joint pain for centuries. It contains compounds called harpagosides that have been shown to reduce pain and improve mobility in people with osteoarthritis.

Cayenne pepper: This spice contains capsaicin, a compound that has been shown to reduce pain and improve mobility in people with osteoarthritis. You can take capsaicin supplements or add cayenne pepper to your food.

White willow bark: This herb contains salicin, a compound similar to aspirin that has been used to treat pain and inflammation for centuries. You can take white willow bark supplements or make a tea with the bark.

Stinging nettle: This herb has been used to treat joint pain and inflammation for centuries. It contains compounds called lectins and histamines that have been shown to reduce pain and improve mobility.

Black cohosh: This herb, native to North America, has been used to treat joint pain and inflammation. It contains compounds called triterpene glycosides that have been shown to reduce pain and improve mobility in people with osteoarthritis.

Capsaicin: As mentioned earlier, capsaicin is a compound found in cayenne pepper that has been shown to reduce pain and improve mobility in people with osteoarthritis. It works by depleting substance P, a chemical involved in transmitting pain signals to the brain. Capsaicin cream or ointment can be applied topically to the affected joint for pain relief.

Arnica: This herb has been used to treat joint pain and inflammation for centuries. It contains compounds called sesquiterpene lactones that have anti-inflammatory properties. Arnica gel or cream can be applied topically to the affected joint for pain relief.

Rosehip: This fruit is a rich source of vitamin C and antioxidants, which have anti-inflammatory properties. Rosehip supplements or oil can be taken or applied topically to help reduce joint pain.

Green-lipped mussel: This shellfish is a rich source of omega-3 fatty acids and other anti-inflammatory compounds. Green-lipped mussel supplements or oil can be taken to help reduce joint pain.

Hyaluronic acid: This compound is found naturally in the body and is a component of synovial fluid, which lubricates the joints. Hyaluronic acid supplements have been shown to reduce pain and improve mobility in people with osteoarthritis.

Collagen: This protein is a major component of cartilage, tendons, and ligaments. Collagen supplements have been shown to reduce pain and improve mobility in people with osteoarthritis and other joint conditions.

MSM: This compound, also known as methylsulfonylmethane, has anti-inflammatory properties and has been used to treat joint pain. MSM supplements are available, or it can be taken as a powder or in capsules.

DMSO: This compound, also known as dimethyl sulfoxide, is a solvent that has been used to treat joint pain and inflammation. DMSO cream or gel can be applied topically to the affected joint for pain relief.

Echinacea: This herb has been used to treat joint pain and inflammation for centuries. It contains compounds called echinacosides that have anti-inflammatory properties. Echinacea supplements or tea can be taken to help reduce joint pain.

Ginkgo biloba: This herb has been used to treat joint pain and inflammation for centuries. It contains compounds called flavonoids and terpenoids that have anti-inflammatory properties. Ginkgo biloba supplements or tea can be taken to help reduce joint pain.

Milk thistle: This herb has been used to treat joint pain and inflammation for centuries. It contains compounds called silymarin and silibinin that have anti-inflammatory properties. Milk thistle supplements or tea can be taken to help reduce joint pain.

Holy basil: This herb has been used to treat joint pain and inflammation for centuries. It contains compounds called eugenol and methyl eugenol that have anti-inflammatory properties. Holy basil supplements or tea can be taken to help reduce joint pain.

Licorice root: This herb has been used to treat joint pain and inflammation for centuries. It contains compounds called glycyrrhizin and flavonoids that have anti-inflammatory properties. Licorice root supplements or tea can be taken to help reduce joint pain.

Wild yam: This herb has been used to treat joint pain and inflammation for centuries. It contains compounds called diosgenin and dioscin that have anti-inflammatory properties. Wild yam supplements or cream can be taken or applied topically to help reduce joint pain.

Birch leaf: This herb has been used to treat joint pain and inflammation for centuries. It contains compounds called methyl salicylate and flavonoids that have anti-inflammatory properties. Birch leaf supplements or tea can be taken to help reduce joint pain.

Nettle leaf: This herb has been used to treat joint pain and inflammation for centuries. It contains compounds called histamine and formic acid that have anti-inflammatory properties. Nettle leaf supplements or tea can be taken to help reduce joint pain.

Yucca root: This herb has been used to treat joint pain and inflammation for centuries. It contains compounds called saponins and steroidal glycosides that have anti-inflammatory properties. Yucca root supplements or tea can be taken to help reduce joint pain.

Calendula: This herb has been used to treat joint pain and inflammation for centuries. It contains compounds called flavonoids and triterpenoids that have anti-inflammatory properties. Calendula supplements or cream can be taken or applied topically to help reduce joint pain.

Sarsaparilla: This herb has been used to treat joint pain and inflammation for centuries. It contains compounds called saponins and steroidal glycosides that have anti-inflammatory properties. Sarsaparilla supplements or tea can be taken to help reduce joint pain.

Dandelion root: This herb has been used to treat joint pain and inflammation for centuries. It contains compounds called flavonoids and triterpenoids that have anti-inflammatory properties. Dandelion root supplements or tea can be taken to help reduce joint pain.

Cat's claw: This herb has been used to treat joint pain and inflammation for centuries. It contains compounds called alkaloids and flavonoids that have anti-inflammatory properties. Cat's claw supplements or tea can be taken to help reduce joint pain.

Garlic: This herb has been used to treat joint pain and inflammation for centuries. It contains compounds called allicin and diallyl disulfide that have anti-inflammatory properties. Garlic supplements or cloves can be taken to help reduce joint pain.

Apple cider vinegar: This liquid has been used to treat joint pain and inflammation for centuries. It contains acetic acid and other compounds that have anti-inflammatory properties. Apple cider vinegar can be taken orally or applied topically to help reduce joint pain.

Lemon juice: This juice has been used to treat joint pain and inflammation for centuries. It contains Vitamin C and other compounds that have anti-inflammatory properties. Lemon juice can be taken orally or applied topically to help reduce joint pain.

Aloe vera: This herb has been used to treat joint pain and inflammation for centuries. It contains compounds called aloin and emodin that have anti-inflammatory properties. Aloe vera gel or cream can be applied topically to the affected joint for pain relief.

Coconut oil: This oil has been used to treat joint pain and inflammation for centuries. It contains medium-chain fatty acids that have anti-inflammatory properties. Coconut oil can be taken orally or applied topically to help reduce joint pain.

Olive oil: This oil has been used to treat joint pain and inflammation for centuries. It contains monounsaturated fatty acids that have anti-inflammatory properties. Olive oil can be taken orally or applied topically to help reduce joint pain.

Flaxseed oil: This oil has been used to treat joint pain and inflammation for centuries. It contains omega-3 fatty acids that have anti-inflammatory properties. Flaxseed oil can be taken orally or applied topically to help reduce joint pain.

Fish oil: This oil has been used to treat joint pain and inflammation for centuries. It contains omega-3 fatty acids that have anti-inflammatory properties. Fish oil supplements can be taken to help reduce joint pain.

Evening primrose oil: This oil has been used to treat joint pain and inflammation for centuries. It contains gamma-linolenic acid that has anti-inflammatory properties. Evening primrose oil supplements can be taken to help reduce joint pain.

Burdock root: This herb has been used to treat joint pain and inflammation for centuries. It contains compounds called inulin and mucilage that have anti-inflammatory properties. Burdock root supplements or tea can be taken to help reduce joint pain.

Red clover: This herb has been used to treat joint pain and inflammation for centuries. It contains compounds called isoflavones that have anti-inflammatory properties. Red clover supplements or tea can be taken to help reduce joint pain.

Meadowsweet: This herb has been used to treat joint pain and inflammation for centuries. It contains compounds called salicylic acid and flavonoids that have anti-inflammatory properties. Meadowsweet supplements or tea can be taken to help reduce joint pain.

Valerian root: This herb has been used to treat joint pain and inflammation for centuries. It contains compounds called valerenic acid and valepotriates that have anti-inflammatory properties. Valerian root supplements or tea can be taken to help reduce joint pain.

Blackcurrant seed oil: This oil has been used to treat joint pain and inflammation for centuries. It contains gamma-linolenic acid and other compounds that have anti-inflammatory properties. Blackcurrant seed oil supplements can be taken to help reduce joint pain.

Celery seed oil: This oil has been used to treat joint pain and inflammation for centuries. It contains compounds called apigenin and luteolin that have anti-inflammatory properties. Celery seed oil can be applied topically to the affected joint for pain relief.

Frankincense oil: This oil has been used to treat joint pain and inflammation for centuries. It contains compounds called boswellic acids that have anti-inflammatory properties. Frankincense oil can be applied topically to the affected joint for pain relief or inhaled for aromatherapy.

Peppermint oil: This oil has been used to treat joint pain and inflammation for centuries. It contains compounds called menthol and menthone that have anti-inflammatory properties. Peppermint oil can be applied topically to the affected joint for pain relief or inhaled for aromatherapy.

Conclusion

It is important to note that these remedies are traditionally used for joint pain and inflammation and have not been scientifically proven to be effective. It is always best to check with a doctor before trying any new treatment. Additionally, some of these remedies may interact with certain medications or have side effects, so it is important to be cautious when using them.

It's also important to note that while these natural remedies may provide some relief for joint pain, they should not be used as a substitute for proper medical care and treatment. If joint pain persists or becomes severe, it is important to consult with a healthcare professional for proper diagnosis and treatment. Additionally, maintaining a healthy diet, regular exercise, and maintaining a healthy weight can all help to alleviate joint pain and inflammation.

In summary, there are many natural remedies that have been traditionally used to alleviate joint pain and inflammation. Some of the most popular remedies include turmeric, ginger, omega-3 fatty acids, boswellia, glucosamine, chondroitin, bromelain, devil's claw, cayenne pepper, white willow bark, stinging nettle, black cohosh, capsaicin, arnica, rosehip, green-lipped mussel, hyaluronic acid, collagen, MSM, DMSO, Echinacea, Ginkgo biloba, Milk thistle, Holy basil, Licorice root, Wild yam, Birch leaf, Nettle leaf, Yucca root, Calendula, Sarsaparilla, Dandelion root, Cat's claw, Garlic, Apple cider vinegar, Lemon juice, Aloe vera, Coconut oil, Olive oil, Flaxseed oil, Fish oil, Evening primrose oil, Burdock root, Red clover,

Meadowsweet, Valerian root, Blackcurrant seed oil, Celery seed oil, Frankincense oil, and Peppermint oil. However, it is always best to check with a doctor before trying any new treatment and to not use them as substitute of proper medical care and treatment.